GALVESTON DIET

MANAGING HORMONAL CHANGES WITH DETERMINATION AND WELL INFORMED GUIDANCE

MARY J. WEBB

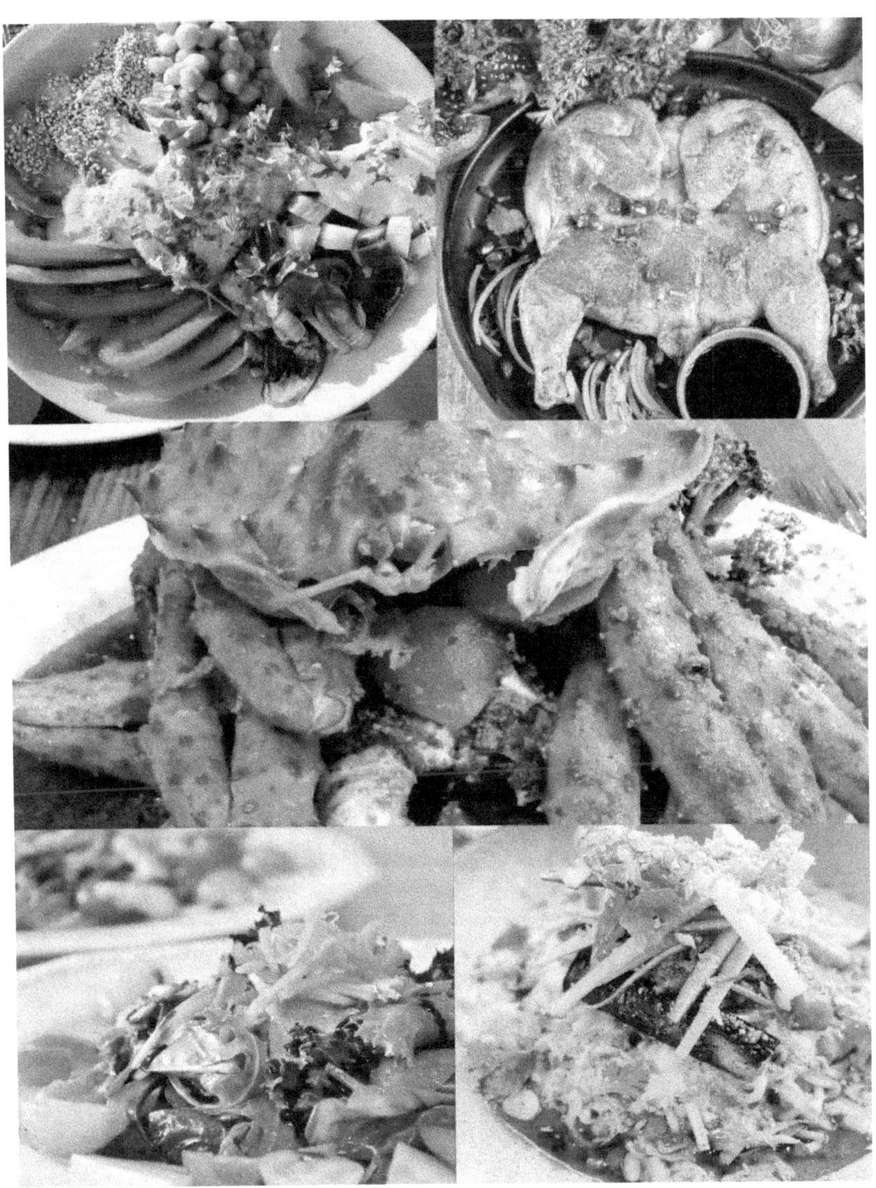

TABLE OF CONTENTS

INTRODUCTION 13

A Galveston Success Story: Sarah's Transformation 14

CHAPTER 1 16

Health Benefits of the Galveston Diet 16

CHAPTER2 21

How Galveston Diet works 21

CHAPTER 3 27

Changes in Your Body 27

Symptoms of Permenopause 28

CHAPTER 4 33

Preparing to Transform Your Life with the Galveston Diet 33

Grasping the Galveston Diet 33

Steps to Get Ready for the Galveston Diet 34

Tips for Success 38

Potential Challenges and Solutions 39

CHAPTER 6 41

Comprehensive Galveston Diet Meal Plan and Shopping Lists 41

Sample 7-Day Meal Plan 41

Day 1: 41

Day 2: 42

Day 3: 42

Day 4: 43

Day 5: 43

Day 6: 44

Day 7: 44

Shopping List 45

1. Proteins: 45

2. Vegetables: 46

3. Fruits: 47

4. Healthy Fats: 47

5. Grains and Legumes: 48

6. Condiments and Snacks: 48

7. Spices and Seasonings: 49

8. Other: 49

Intermittent Fasting Guidelines 50

Tips: 50

CHAPTER 7 51

Comprehensive 30-Day Galveston Diet Meal Plan with Recipes. 51

Week 1 51

Day 1: 51

Breakfast: 51

Lunch: 52

Snack: 52

Dinner: 52

Day 2: 53

Breakfast: 53

Lunch: 53

Snack: 54

Dinner: 54

Day 3: 55

Breakfast: 55

Lunch: 55

Snack: 55

Dinner: 56

Day 4: 56

Breakfast: 56

Lunch: 56

Snack: 57

Dinner: 57

Day 5: 58

Breakfast: 58

Lunch: 58

Snack: 59

Dinner: 59

Day 6: 60

Breakfast: 60

Lunch: 60

Snack: 61

Day 7: 61

Breakfast: 61

Lunch: 61

Snack: 62

Dinner: 62

Week 2 63

Day 8: 63

Breakfast: 63

Lunch: 63

Snack: 64

Dinner: 64

Day 9: 65

Breakfast: 65

Lunch: 65

Snack: 65

Dinner: 66

Day 10: 66

Breakfast: 66

Lunch: 67

Snack: 67

Dinner: 67

Day 11: 68

Breakfast: 68

Lunch: 68

Snack: 69

Dinner: 69

Day 12: 70

Breakfast: 70

Lunch: 70

Snack: 71

Dinner: 71

Day 13: 72

Breakfast: 72

Lunch: 72

Dinner: 73

Day 14: 74

Breakfast: 74

Lunch: 74

Snack: 74

Dinner: 75

WEEK 3 76

Day 15: 76

Breakfast: 76

Lunch: 76

Snack: 76

Dinner: 77

Day 16: 77

Breakfast: 77

Lunch: 77

Snack: 78

Dinner: 78

Day 17: 79

Breakfast: 79

Lunch: 79

Snack: 79

Dinner: 80

Day 18: 80

Breakfast: 80

Lunch: 80

Snack: 81

Dinner: 81

Day 19: 82

Breakfast: 82

Lunch: 82

Snack: 82

Dinner: 83

Day 20: 84

Breakfast: 84

Lunch: 84

Snack: 84

Dinner: 85

Day 21: 86

Breakfast: 86

Lunch: 86

Snack: 86

Dinner: 87

WEEK 4 88

Day 22: 88

Breakfast: 88

Lunch: 88

Snack: 88

Dinner: 89

Day 23: 89

Breakfast: 89

Lunch: 90

Snack: 90

Dinner: 90

Day 24: 91

Breakfast: 91

Lunch: 91

Snack: 92

Dinner: 92

Day 25: 93

Breakfast: 93

Lunch: 93

Snack: 93

Dinner: 94

Day 26: 94

Breakfast: 94

Lunch: 94

Snack: 95

Dinner: 95

Day 27: 96

Breakfast: 96

Lunch: 96

Snack: 96

Dinner: 97

Day 28: 97

Breakfast: 97

Lunch: 98

Snack: 98

Dinner: 98

Day 29: 99

Breakfast: 99

Lunch: 99

Snack: 99

Dinner: 100

Day 30: 101

Breakfast: 101

Lunch: 101

Snack: 101

Dinner: 102

CHAPTER 8 103

Galveston Diet Glossary 103

CHAPTER 9 108

CONCLUSION 108

INTRODUCTION

In today's health-conscious world, finding a sustainable and effective diet can be challenging.

Enter the Galveston Diet, a beacon of hope for those seeking not just weight loss but a comprehensive lifestyle change. Created by Mary J. Webb, the Galveston Diet transcends calorie counting and restrictive eating, emphasizing anti-inflammatory principles, intermittent fasting, and nutrient-rich foods.

This diet is scientifically supported and tailored for women, especially those in midlife, to reclaim their health and vitality. It addresses often-ignored aspects of weight management like hormonal balance and inflammation, offering a holistic wellness approach. It's crafted to help women through menopause, premenopausal, and beyond, providing a sustainable path to long-term health.

A Galveston Success Story: Sarah's Transformation

Sarah, a 52-year-old mother of two, had struggled with weight, fatigue, and mood swings for years. Desperate for a solution, she discovered the Galveston Diet. Intrigued by its focus on anti-inflammatory foods and intermittent fasting, she decided to try it.

Within weeks, Sarah's energy levels soared, her stubborn midsection weight began to melt away, and her mood stabilized. Beyond physical changes, Sarah regained control over her health and life, finding support in a community of women facing similar challenges. The Galveston Diet transformed her mindset and relationship with food.

Today, Sarah is a proud advocate of the Galveston Diet. She has maintained her weight loss and embraced a lifestyle that continues to support her well-being. Sarah's story is one of many, illustrating the profound impact of the Galveston Diet.

The Galveston Diet is more than a diet; it's a movement towards a healthier, happier life. Whether dealing with weight management, hormonal imbalances, or seeking a sustainable way to improve well-being, the Galveston Diet offers a science-based, compassionate approach. Join us on this transformative journey and discover the power of the Galveston Diet for yourself.

CHAPTER 1

Health Benefits of the Galveston Diet

The Galveston Diet offers numerous health benefits, particularly for women in midlife. Here are some advantages.

1. Weight Loss and Management

Consistent Weight Loss: The diet promotes steady and sustainable weight loss through intermittent fasting, reduced carbohydrate intake, and anti-inflammatory foods.

Decreased Abdominal Fat: By stabilizing blood sugar and enhancing metabolic health, the diet targets stubborn belly fat.

2. Hormonal Balance

Relief from Menopausal Symptoms: The diet helps balance hormones, reducing common menopausal symptoms like hot flashes, night sweats, and mood swings.

Enhanced Insulin Sensitivity: Intermittent fasting and lower carbohydrate intake improve insulin sensitivity, essential for hormonal balance.

3. Reduced Inflammation

Chronic Disease Prevention: Anti-inflammatory foods lower the risk of chronic diseases such as heart disease, diabetes, and certain cancers.

Pain and Discomfort Reduction: Lowering inflammation can alleviate symptoms of inflammatory conditions like arthritis and other joint issues.

4. Improved Metabolic Health

Better Blood Sugar Control: Emphasizing low-glycemic foods and intermittent fasting helps stabilize blood sugar levels, reducing the risk of diabetes.

Enhanced Fat Utilization: Intermittent fasting improves the body's ability to burn fat for energy, boosting metabolic efficiency.

5. Increased Energy Levels

Sustained Energy: Balanced blood sugar and nutrient-dense foods provide steady energy throughout the day, reducing fatigue and increasing overall vitality.

Better Sleep Quality: Hormonal balance and reduced inflammation contribute to improved sleep patterns and quality.

6. Enhanced Mental Clarity and Mood

Better Cognitive Function: Stabilized blood sugar and a balanced diet support brain health, improving focus, memory, and mental clarity.

Mood Stability: Balanced hormones and reduced inflammation lead to more stable moods and a lower risk of depression and anxiety.

7. Better Digestive Health

Regular Bowel Movements: A fiber-rich diet from vegetables, fruits, and whole grains promotes healthy digestion and regularity.

Gut Health: Anti-inflammatory foods support a healthy gut micro biome, essential for overall digestive health and immune function.

8. Cardiovascular Health

Lower Cholesterol Levels: Healthy fats and fiber-rich foods help reduce bad cholesterol (LDL) and increase good cholesterol (HDL).

Reduced Blood Pressure: Anti-inflammatory nutrition and regular physical activity contribute to healthier blood pressure levels.

9. Longevity and Quality of Life

Healthy Aging: The diet's focus on nutrient-dense foods, hormonal balance, and inflammation reduction supports healthy aging and longevity.

Improved Quality of Life: Enhanced physical health, mental clarity, and emotional well-being lead to a better overall quality of life.

The Galveston Diet provides a comprehensive approach to health, addressing multiple aspects of well-being. By focusing on sustainable weight management, hormonal balance, reduced inflammation, improved metabolic health, and overall vitality, it offers a holistic path to better health and longevity for women in midlife.

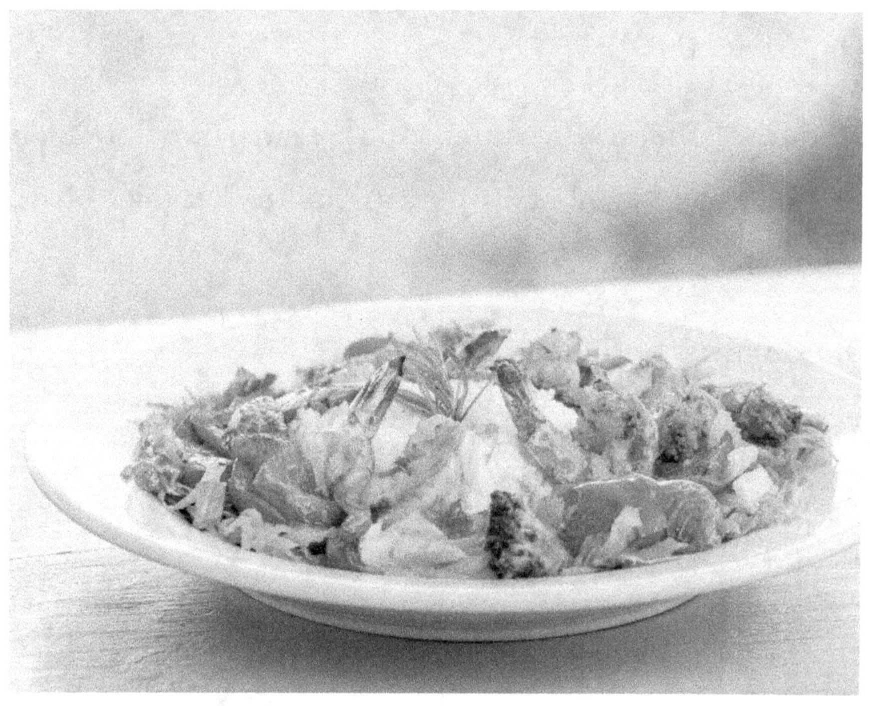

CHAPTER 2

How Galveston Diet works

The Galveston Diet is built on a unique combination of strategies that cater specifically to the needs of women, particularly those in midlife. Here are the main strategies that define the Galveston Diet:

1. Anti-Inflammatory Nutrition

The Galveston Diet prioritizes foods that help reduce inflammation in the body, as chronic inflammation is linked to numerous health problems, including weight gain and metabolic disorders. The diet focuses on:

Healthy Fats: Incorporating sources such as avocados, nuts, seeds, and olive oil to decrease inflammation and enhance heart health.

Lean Proteins: Including options like fish, poultry, and plant-based proteins to support muscle maintenance and overall health.

Fiber-Rich Foods: Consuming a variety of vegetables, fruits, and whole grains to support digestive health and provide essential nutrients.

2. Intermittent Fasting

Intermittent fasting (IF) is a core component of the Galveston Diet. IF involves alternating periods of eating and fasting, which can help regulate hormones, boost metabolism, and aid in weight loss. Popular methods include:

16/8 Method: Fasting for 16 hours and eating all meals within an 8-hour window.

5:2 Method: Eating normally for five days a week and reducing calories to about 500-600 on the other two days.

3. Carbohydrate Reduction

Cutting down on carbohydrate intake, particularly refined carbs and sugars, is essential in the Galveston Diet. This helps stabilize blood sugar levels and prevent insulin spikes.

The focus is on:

Low-Glycemic Foods: Choosing carbs that have a lower impact on blood sugar, such as non-starchy vegetables, berries, and legumes.

Whole Foods: Prioritizing unprocessed foods over refined and processed options.

4. Hormonal Balance

The Galveston Diet addresses hormonal imbalances that often affect women in midlife, helping to alleviate symptoms like weight gain, fatigue, and mood swings. Strategies include:

Phytoestrogens: Including foods like flaxseeds, soy, and certain vegetables to help balance estrogen levels.

Nutrient-Dense Foods: Ensuring adequate intake of vitamins and minerals that support hormonal health, such as vitamin D, magnesium, and omega-3 fatty acids.

5. Mindful Eating

The Galveston Diet encourages mindful eating practices to help individuals become more aware of their hunger and fullness cues, leading to healthier eating habits and a better relationship with food. This involves:

Eating Slowly: Taking time to enjoy meals and recognize when you're full.

Avoiding Distractions: Focusing on eating without distractions like screens or multitasking.

6. Regular Physical Activity

While diet plays a significant role, incorporating regular physical activity is also crucial. Exercise helps boost metabolism, maintain muscle mass, and improve overall well-being. Recommendations include:

Strength Training: Building and maintaining muscle through resistance exercises.

Cardiovascular Exercise: Engaging in activities like walking, running, or cycling to improve heart health and burn calories.

Flexibility and Balance: Including activities like yoga or stretching to enhance flexibility and prevent injuries.

7. Community and Support

The Galveston Diet highlights the importance of community and support. Joining a group of like-minded individuals can provide motivation, accountability, and a sense of belonging. This can be done through:

Online Communities: Participating in forums, social media groups, or online classes.

Local Groups: Engaging with local health clubs, support groups, or fitness classes.

These strategies create a holistic approach to health and wellness, making the Galveston Diet a comprehensive plan tailored to the needs of women in midlife. By focusing on anti-inflammatory nutrition, intermittent fasting, carbohydrate reduction, hormonal balance, mindful eating, regular physical activity, and community support, the Galveston Diet provides a sustainable path to long-term health and vitality.

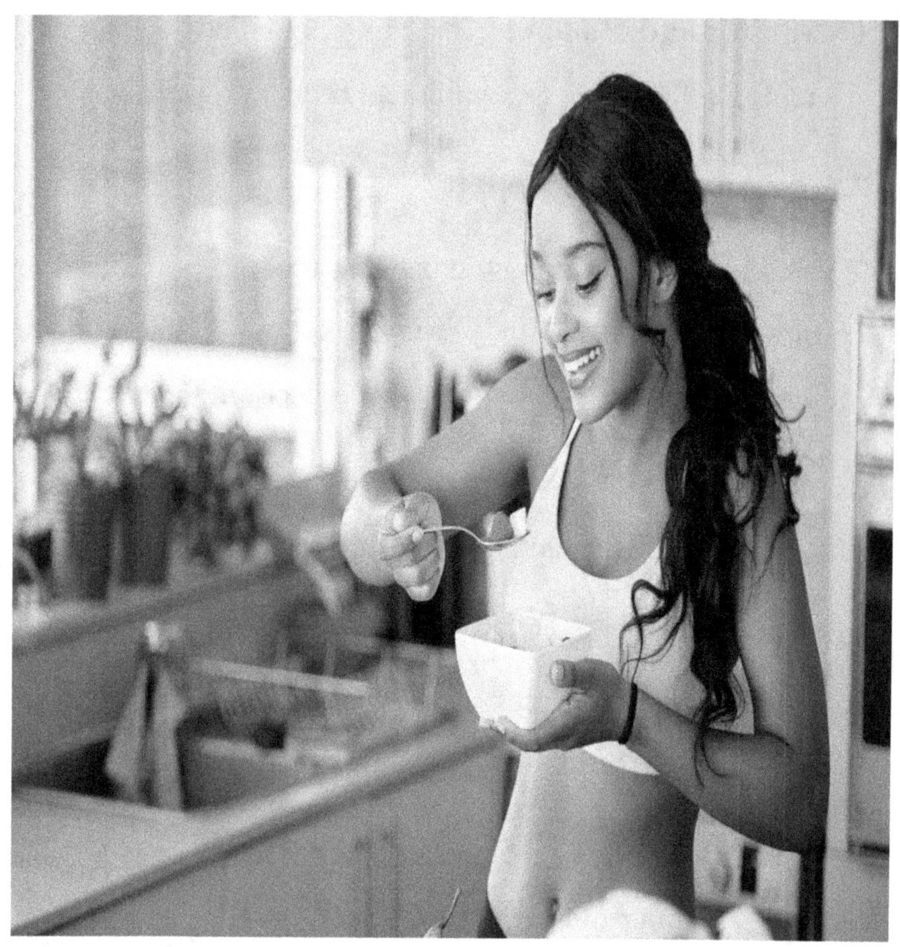

CHAPTER 3

Changes in Your Body

Premenopause

Premenopause, also called the menopausal transition, is the period leading up to menopause marked by hormonal changes and a gradual decline in reproductive function. This phase usually begins in a woman's 40s but can start earlier and can last for several years. During premenopause, the ovaries produce less estrogen and progesterone, leading to irregular menstrual cycles, changes in menstrual flow, and eventually the cessation of menstruation. Symptoms of premenopause can vary widely among women but commonly include hot flashes, night sweats, mood swings, sleep disturbances, and vaginal dryness. Other possible symptoms include weight gain, thinning hair, dry skin, and decreased libido. Hormonal fluctuations during this time can also affect bone density and cardiovascular health. It is important for women experiencing premenopause to maintain a healthy lifestyle, including a balanced diet, regular exercise, and routine medical checkups to manage symptoms and monitor their health. Healthcare providers may recommend treatments such as hormone replacement therapy (HRT) or non-hormonal options to alleviate severe symptoms. Understanding and recognizing the signs of premenopause can help women better prepare for the changes associated with this natural stage of aging.

Symptoms of Permenopause

1. Hot Flashes and Night Sweats

Hot Flashes: Sudden sensations of warmth, usually affecting the face, neck, and chest, often leading to sweating and discomfort. They can vary in intensity and duration, often followed by a chill.

Night Sweats: Intense sweating during sleep, sometimes severe enough to soak through clothing and bedding, disrupting sleep and causing fatigue.

2. Menstrual Irregularities

Irregular Periods: Variations in the length, flow, and frequency of menstrual cycles. Periods may become lighter, heavier, or irregular as hormone levels fluctuate.

Spotting: Unpredictable light bleeding between periods.

3. Mood Changes

Mood Swings: Rapid shifts in mood, ranging from happiness to irritability or sadness, often without an obvious cause.

Anxiety and Depression: Increased levels of anxiety or depression. Some women may experience panic attacks or heightened stress.

Irritability: Increased sensitivity to stress, leading to easy annoyance or frustration.

4. Sleep Disturbances

Insomnia: Difficulty falling asleep, staying asleep, or waking up too early, often due to night sweats or other hormonal changes.

Restless Sleep: Frequent awakenings during the night without clear reasons.

5. Vaginal and Urinary Symptoms

Vaginal Dryness: Reduced lubrication, causing discomfort, itching, or burning in the vaginal area.

Discomfort During Intercourse: Painful or uncomfortable sexual activity due to vaginal dryness and thinning of the vaginal walls.

Urinary Issues: Increased frequency, urgency, or a higher risk of urinary tract infections (UTIs).

6. Physical Changes

Weight Gain: Often around the abdomen, due to changes in metabolism and hormone levels.

Thinning Hair and Dry Skin: Changes in hair texture and volume, along with increased skin dryness.

Breast Tenderness: Swelling and soreness in the breasts, similar to premenstrual symptoms.

Joint and Muscle Pain: General aches and stiffness, particularly in the mornings.

7. Sexual Changes

Decreased Libido: Reduced interest in sex, potentially due to hormonal changes, physical discomfort, or emotional factors.

Changes in Sexual Response: Alterations in arousal, response, and satisfaction during sexual activity.

8. Cognitive Symptoms

Brain Fog: Difficulties with concentration, memory lapses, and a general sense of mental sluggishness.

Forgetfulness: More frequent memory lapses or difficulty recalling names, dates, and other information.

9. Other Symptoms

Fatigue: Persistent tiredness or low energy, not necessarily related to sleep quality.

Headaches: Increased frequency or intensity of headaches, which may be linked to hormonal fluctuations.

Digestive Changes: Bloating, changes in bowel habits, or other digestive issues.

Understanding these symptoms and their potential impact on daily life can help women seek appropriate medical advice and support during premenopause. Managing lifestyle factors such as diet, exercise, stress, and sleep hygiene can help alleviate some symptoms, while medical treatments may be necessary for others.

CHAPTER 4

Preparing to Transform Your Life with the Galveston Diet

The Galveston Diet, developed by Dr. Mary J. Webb, targets women in midlife to combat weight gain and health issues linked to menopause. It emphasizes anti-inflammatory foods, intermittent fasting, and a low carbohydrate intake. Here's a comprehensive guide to help you prepare for and thrive on the Galveston Diet.

Grasping the Galveston Diet

Core Concepts:

1. Anti-Inflammatory Foods: Focus on foods that reduce inflammation.

2. Intermittent Fasting: Integrate fasting periods to enhance metabolism and hormonal balance.

3. Low Carbohydrate Intake: Minimize carbohydrate intake to manage insulin levels and encourage fat loss.

Steps to Get Ready for the Galveston Diet

1. Educate Yourself:

Read Mary J. Webb's book or other reliable sources on the Galveston Diet.

2. Learn about the diet's science and benefits.

Consult a Healthcare Professional:

3. Discuss your plans with your doctor, especially if you already have existing health conditions.

Ensure the diet is safe and suitable for your personal needs.

4. Set clear goals:

Identify what you want to achieve (e.g., weight loss, increased energy, better hormonal balance).

Establish realistic, measurable goals to track your progress.

5. Plan Your Meals:

Develop a weekly meal plan featuring a variety of anti-inflammatory foods.

Make a shopping list with the necessary ingredients to avoid last-minute unhealthy choices.

6. Understanding Intermittent Fasting:

Choose a fasting window that fits your lifestyle (e.g., 16/8, 18/6).

Start gradually if you are new to fasting, lengthening the fasting period over time.

7. Stock Your Kitchen:

Remove processed and high-carb foods from your pantry.

Stock up on healthy fats, lean proteins, vegetables, and low-glycemic fruits.

Implementing the Galveston Diet

8. Anti-Inflammatory Foods:

Include: Fatty fish (salmon, mackerel), leafy greens (spinach, kale), nuts and seeds, olive oil, berries, and turmeric.

Avoid processed foods, sugary snacks, refined carbohydrates, and Tran's fats.

9. Intermittent Fasting:

Start: Begin with a 12-hour fast and gradually increase to 16-18 hours.

Hydrate: Drink plenty of water, herbal teas, and black coffee during the fasting window.

Break the fast: Start with a balanced meal that includes protein, healthy fats, and vegetables.

10. Low Carbohydrate Intake:

Focus on non-starchy vegetables, low-glycemic fruits, and healthy fats.

Limit: bread, pasta, rice, and sugary foods.

11. Exercise:

Incorporate regular physical activity into your routine, such as walking, yoga, jogging, or strength training.

Aim for 150 minutes of moderate aerobic activities.

12. Monitor Progress:

Keep a food journal to track your meals, fasting periods, and any changes in your health.

13. Use apps or tools to monitor your progress and stay motivated.

1. Stay Hydrated:

Drink at least 8 glasses of water a day.

Consider adding electrolytes if you feel fatigued.

2. Support System:

Share your journey with friends or family members.

Join online communities or groups following the Galveston Diet for support and motivation.

3. Be Flexible:

Listen to your body and adjust your fasting and meal plans as needed.

Don't be too hard on yourself if you slip up; focus on consistency rather than perfection.

4. Educate yourself continuously.

Stay informed about new research and updates related to the Galveston Diet.

Experiment with new recipes and meal ideas to keep the diet enjoyable.

Potential Challenges and Solutions

1. Hunger during Fasting:

Solution: Start with shorter fasting periods and gradually increase according to your strength. Drink water or herbal tea to curb your hunger.

2. Cravings for Carbs:

Solution: Include healthy fats and proteins in your meals to stay satiated. Keep low-carb snacks handy.

3. Social Situations:

Solution: Plan ahead for social events by checking menus in advance. Communicate your dietary needs to friends and family members.

4. Plateaus:

Solution: Reassess your meal plan and fasting schedule. Consider varying your exercise routine to boost metabolism.

Preparing for and following the Galveston Diet involves understanding its principles, planning your meals, and incorporating lifestyle changes like intermittent fasting and regular exercise. By educating yourself, setting clear goals, and staying flexible, you can successfully transition to this diet and achieve your health goals. Remember to consult with a healthcare professional before making any significant dietary changes, and listen to your body throughout the process.

CHAPTER 6

Comprehensive Galveston Diet Meal Plan and Shopping Lists

The Galveston Diet focuses on anti-inflammatory foods, balanced macronutrients, intermittent fasting, and low carbohydrate intake. Here's a detailed meal plan and shopping list to help you embark on this dietary approach.

Sample 7-Day Meal Plan

Day 1:

Breakfast: Greek yogurt garnished with berries and chia seeds

Lunch: Grilled salmon salad with mixed greens, cherry tomatoes, avocado, and olive oil dressing

Snack: Handful of almonds

Dinner: Baked chicken breast with steamed broccoli and cauliflower rice

Day 2:

Breakfast: Smoothie with spinach, avocado, berries, and almond milk

Lunch: Turkey and avocado lettuce wraps with a side of carrot sticks

Snack: Sliced cucumber with hummus

Dinner: Shrimp stir-fry with bell peppers, zucchini, and quinoa

Day 3:

Breakfast: Scrambled eggs, spinach and feta cheese

Lunch: Tuna salad, mixed greens, olives, and a lemon vinaigrette

Snack: Apple slices with almond butter

Dinner: Grilled steak with asparagus and a side salad

Breakfast: Chia seed pudding with coconut milk and fresh berries

Lunch: Quinoa and black bean salad with cilantro and lime dressing

Snack: Mixed nuts

Dinner: Baked cod with sautéed kale and sweet potato mash

Day 5:

Breakfast: Ouellette with tomatoes, mushrooms, and spinach

Lunch: Chicken Caesar salad (with olive oil and lemon dressing)

Snack: Bell pepper slices with guacamole

Dinner: Turkey meatballs, zucchini noodles and marinara sauce

Day 6:

Breakfast: Greek yogurt with walnuts and a drizzle of honey

Lunch: Mixed greens with grilled chicken, avocado, and balsamic vinaigrette

Snack: Blueberries and a few pieces of dark chocolate

Dinner: Grilled salmon, roasted Brussels sprouts and quinoa

Day 7:

Breakfast: Smoothie with kale, banana, almond butter, and flaxseeds

Lunch: Spinach and feta stuffed bell peppers

Snack: Handful of pumpkin seeds

Dinner: Grilled pork chops with green beans and mashed cauliflower

1. Proteins:

Chicken breast

Salmon fillets

Shrimp

Tuna

Turkey breast

Cod fillets

Steak

Ground turkey

Pork chops

Greek yogurt

Eggs

2. Vegetables:

Spinach

Mixed greens

Cherry tomatoes

Avocado

Broccoli

Cauliflower

Bell peppers

Zucchini

Asparagus

Kale

Sweet potatoes

Mushrooms

Cucumbers

Carrots

Brussels sprouts

Green beans

3. Fruits:

Berries (blueberries, strawberries, and raspberries)

Apples

Bananas

Avocado

Lemons

4. Healthy Fats:

Olive oil

Avocado

Nuts (almonds, walnuts)

Seeds (chia seeds, flaxseeds, pumpkin seeds)

Almond butter

Coconut milk

5. Grains and Legumes:

Quinoa

Black beans

6. Condiments and Snacks:

Hummus

Guacamole

Dark chocolate (70% cacao or higher)

Mixed nuts

Herbal teas

Almond milk

7. Spices and Seasonings:

Salt

Black pepper

Turmeric

Cumin Paprika

Garlic powder

Onion powder

Dried herbs (basil, oregano, thyme)

8. Other:

Chia seeds

Flaxseeds

Honey (for drizzling)

Intermittent Fasting Guidelines

♣ Typical Fasting Windows:

16/8: Fast for 16 hours, eat within an 8-hour window.

18/6: Fast for 18 hours; eat within a 6-hour window most times.

Tips:

♣ **Hydration:** Drink enough water, herbal teas, and black coffee during fasting periods.

♣ **Gradual Start:** If new to fasting, start with shorter fasting periods and gradually extend them.

♣ **Meal Timing:** Break your fast with a balanced meal that includes protein, healthy fats, and vegetable

CHAPTER 7

Comprehensive 30-Day Galveston Diet Meal Plan with Recipes.

The Galveston Diet focuses on anti-inflammatory foods, balanced macronutrients, intermittent fasting, and low carbohydrate intake. Below is a 30-day meal plan complete with recipes and preparation methods.

Week 1

Day 1:

Breakfast: Greek Yogurt with Berries and Chia Seeds

Ingredients: 1 cup Greek yogurt, 1/2 cup mixed berries, and 1 tablespoon chia seeds.

Preparation: Combine Greek yogurt, berries, and chia seeds in a bowl. Let it sit for 5 minutes to allow the chia seeds to absorb moisture.

Lunch: **Grilled Salmon Salad**

Ingredients: 1 salmon fillet, 2 cups mixed greens, 1/2 cup cherry tomatoes, 1/2 avocado, 1 tbsp. olive oil, 1 tbsp. lemon juice, salt, and pepper.

Preparation: Grill the salmon until fully cooked. Toss mixed greens, cherry tomatoes, and avocado with olive oil, lemon juice, salt, and pepper. Top with the grilled salmon.

Snack: **Handful of Almonds**

Ingredients: 1/4 cup almonds.

Dinner: Baked Chicken Breast with Steamed Broccoli and Cauliflower Rice

Ingredients: 1 chicken breast, 1 cup broccoli florets, 1 cup cauliflower rice, 1 tablespoon olive oil, salt, and pepper.

Preparation: Preheat the oven to 375°F (190°C). Season the chicken with salt and pepper, and bake for 25–30 minutes until cooked. Steam the broccoli and sauté the cauliflower rice in olive oil for 5–7 minutes.

Day 2:

Breakfast: Spinach, Avocado, and Berry Smoothie

Ingredients: 1 cup spinach, 1/2 avocado, 1/2 cup mixed berries, and 1 cup almond milk.

Preparation: Blend all ingredients until smooth.

Lunch: Turkey and Avocado Lettuce Wraps with Carrot Sticks

Ingredients: 4 large lettuce leaves, 4 slices turkey breast, 1/2 avocado (sliced), 1 cup carrot sticks.

Preparation: Lay turkey slices and avocado on lettuce leaves and roll up. Serve with carrot sticks.

Snack: Sliced Cucumber with Hummus

Ingredients: 1 cucumber, 1/4 cup hummus.

Preparation: Slice the cucumber and enjoy with hummus.

Dinner: Shrimp Stir-Fry with Bell Peppers, Zucchini, and Quinoa

Ingredients: 1 cup quinoa, 1 tbsp. olive oil, 1/2 lb. shrimp, 1 bell pepper (sliced), 1 zucchini (sliced), 2 tbsp. soy sauce.

Preparation: Cook quinoa according to package instructions. Heat olive oil in a pan, add shrimp, bell pepper, and zucchini, and sauté until shrimp is cooked. Serve over quinoa with soy sauce.

Day 3:

Breakfast: Scrambled Eggs with Spinach and Feta

Ingredients: 2 eggs, 1 cup spinach, 1/4 cup feta cheese, salt, and pepper.

Preparation: Scramble the eggs in a pan, add spinach, and cook until wilted, then stir in feta.

Lunch: Tuna Salad with Mixed Greens, Olives, and Lemon Vinaigrette

Ingredients: 1 can tuna, 2 cups mixed greens, 1/4 cup olives, 1 tbsp. olive oil, 1 tbsp. lemon juice, salt, and pepper.

Preparation: Combine tuna with olives and mixed greens. Dress with olive oil, lemon juice, salt, and pepper.

Snack: Apple Slices with Almond Butter

Ingredients: 1 apple, 2 tablespoons of almond butter.

Preparation: Slice the apple and serve with almond butter.

Dinner: Grilled Steak with Asparagus and Side Salad

Ingredients: 1 steak, 1 cup asparagus, 2 cups mixed greens, 1/2 cup cherry tomatoes, 1 tbsp. olive oil, 1 tbsp. balsamic vinegar, salt, and pepper.

Preparation: Grill steak to desired doneness. Steam or grill asparagus. Toss mixed greens and cherry tomatoes with olive oil, balsamic vinegar, salt, and pepper.

Day 4:

Breakfast: Chia Seed Pudding with Coconut Milk and Fresh Berries

Ingredients: 1/4 cup chia seeds, 1 cup coconut milk, and 1/2 cup fresh berries.

Preparation: Combine chia seeds and coconut milk; refrigerate overnight. Top with berries before serving.

Lunch: Quinoa and Black Bean Salad with Cilantro and Lime Dressing

Ingredients: 1 cup cooked quinoa, 1 cup black beans, 1/2 cup corn, 1/2 cup cherry tomatoes, 1/4 cup cilantro, 1 tbsp olive oil, 1 tbsp. lime juice, salt, and pepper.

Preparation: Mix quinoa, black beans, corn, cherry tomatoes, and cilantro. Dress with oil, lime juice, salt, and pepper.

Snack: Mixed Nuts

Ingredients: 1/4 cup mixed nuts.

Dinner: Baked Cod with Sautéed Kale and Sweet Potato Mash

Ingredients: 1 cod fillet, 1 cup kale, 1 sweet potato, 1 tablespoon olive oil, salt, and pepper.

Preparation: Preheat the oven to 375°F (190°C). Season the cod with salt and pepper, bake for 15-20 minutes. Sauté kale in olive oil until wilted. Boil and mash sweet potatoes, seasoning with salt and pepper.

Day 5:

Breakfast: Ouellette with Tomatoes, Mushrooms, and Spinach

Ingredients: 2 eggs, 1/2 cup diced tomatoes, 1/2 cup sliced mushrooms, 1 cup spinach, salt, and pepper.

Preparation: Whisk eggs and pour into a heated pan. Add tomatoes, mushrooms, and spinach, cooking until eggs are set.

Lunch: Chicken Caesar Salad (with Olive Oil and Lemon Dressing)

Ingredients: 1 chicken breast, 2 cups romaine lettuce, 1/4 cup grated Parmesan, 1 tbsp. olive oil, 1 tbsp. lemon juice, salt, and pepper.

Preparation: Grill or bake chicken breast. Toss romaine with Parmesan, olive oil, lemon juice, salt, and pepper. Top with sliced chicken.

 Bell Pepper Slices with Guacamole

Ingredients: 1 bell pepper, 1/4 cup guacamole.

Preparation: Slice bell pepper and serve with guacamole.

Dinner: Turkey Meatballs with Zucchini Noodles and Marinara Sauce

Ingredients: 1 lb. ground turkey, 1 egg, 1/4 cup almond flour, 1/4 cup grated Parmesan, 2 zucchinis, 1 cup marinara sauce, 1 tbsp. olive oil, salt, and pepper.

Preparation: Preheat the oven to 375°F (190°C). Mix turkey, egg, almond flour, Parmesan, salt, and pepper; form meatballs and bake for 20-25 minutes. Spiralize zucchinis, sauté in olive oil for 3-5 minutes, and serve meatballs over zucchini noodles with marinara.

Breakfast: Greek Yogurt with Walnuts and Honey

Ingredients: 1 cup Greek yogurt, 1/4 cup walnuts, and 1 tablespoon honey.

Preparation: Top Greek yogurt with walnuts and drizzle with honey.

Lunch: Mixed Greens with Grilled Chicken, Avocado, and Balsamic Vinaigrette

Ingredients: 1 chicken breast, 2 cups mixed greens, 1/2 avocado, 1 tbsp. olive oil, 1 tbsp. balsamic vinegar, salt, and pepper.

Preparation: Grill chicken breast. Toss mixed greens, avocado, olive oil, balsamic vinegar, salt, and pepper, then top with sliced chicken.

Snack: Blueberries and dark chocolate

Ingredients: 1/2 cup blueberries, 1 oz. dark chocolate (70% cacao or higher).

Day 7:

Breakfast: Smoothie with Kale, Banana, Almond Butter, and Flaxseeds

Ingredients: 1 cup kale, 1 banana, 1 tablespoon almond butter, 1 tablespoon flaxseeds, and 1 cup almond milk.

Preparation: Blend all together until smooth.

Lunch: Spinach and Feta Stuffed Bell Peppers

Ingredients: 2 bell peppers, 1 cup spinach, 1/2 cup feta cheese.

Preparation: Preheat the oven to 375°F (190°C). Remove the seeds from the bell peppers. Sauté the spinach, combine it with feta cheese, fill the peppers with the mixture, and bake for 20-25 minutes.

Snack: Pumpkin Seeds

Ingredients: 1/4 cup pumpkin seeds.

Dinner: Grilled Pork Chops with Green Beans

Ingredients: 1 pork chop, 1 cup green beans, 1 head of cauliflower.

Preparation: Grill the pork chop to your preferred doneness. Steam the green beans. Boil the cauliflower, then mash it and season to taste.

Week 2

Breakfast: Greek Yogurt with Berries and Chia Seeds

Ingredients: 1 cup Greek yogurt, 1/2 cup mixed berries, and 1 tablespoon chia seeds.

Preparation: Mix the Greek yogurt, berries, and chia seeds together. Let sit for 5 minutes to allow chia seeds to absorb some moisture.

Lunch: Grilled Chicken Salad with the Greens, Cherry Tomatoes, Avocado, and Olive Oil Dressing

Ingredients: 1 chicken breast, 2 cups mixed greens, 1/2 cup cherry tomatoes, 1/2 avocado, 1 tbsp. olive oil, 1 tbsp. lemon juice, salt and pepper to taste.

Preparation: Grill the chicken breast until cooked through. Toss the mixed greens, cherry tomatoes, and avocado with olive oil, lemon juice, salt, and pepper. Top with grilled chicken.

Snack: **Handful of Walnuts**

Ingredients: 1/4 cup walnuts.

Dinner: Baked Salmon, Steamed Broccoli and Quinoa

Ingredients: 1 salmon fillet, 1 cup broccoli florets, 1 cup quinoa, 1 tablespoon olive oil, salt and pepper to taste.

Preparation: Preheat oven to 375°F (190°C). Season the salmon fillet with salt and pepper, then bake for 15-20 minutes. Steam the broccoli. Cook quinoa according to package instructions.

Breakfast: Smoothie with Spinach, Avocado, Berries, and Almond Milk

Ingredients: 1 cup spinach, 1/2 avocado, 1/2 cup mixed berries, and 1 cup almond milk.

Preparation: Blend all ingredients until smooth.

Lunch: Turkey and Avocado Lettuce Wraps with Celery Sticks

Ingredients: 4 large lettuce leaves, 4 slices turkey breast, 1/2 avocado (sliced), 1 cup celery sticks.

Preparation: Place turkey slices and avocado on lettuce leaves and roll up. Serve with celery sticks.

Snack: Sliced Bell Peppers with Hummus

Ingredients: 1 bell pepper, 1/4 cup hummus.

Preparation: Slice the bell pepper and serve with hummus.

Dinner: **Shrimp Stir-Fry with Bell Peppers, Zucchini, and Quinoa**

Ingredients: 1 cup quinoa, 1 tbsp. olive oil, 1/2 lb. shrimp, 1 bell pepper (sliced), 1 zucchini (sliced), 2 tbsp. soy sauce.

Preparation: Cook quinoa according to package instructions. Heat olive oil in a pan, add shrimp, bell pepper, and zucchini, and sauté until shrimp is cooked. Add soy sauce and serve over quinoa.

Day 10:

Breakfast: **Scrambled Eggs with Kale and Feta Cheese**

Ingredients: 2 eggs, 1 cup kale, 1/4 cup feta cheese, salt and pepper to taste.

Preparation: Scramble the eggs in a pan, add kale and cook until wilted, then stir in feta cheese.

Lunch: Tuna Salad with Mixed Greens, Olives, and Lemon Vinaigrette

Ingredients: 1 can tuna, 2 cups mixed greens, 1/4 cup olives, 1 tablespoon olive oil, 1 tablespoon lemon juice, salt and pepper to taste.

Preparation: Mix tuna with olives and mixed greens. Dress with olive oil, lemon juice, salt, and pepper.

Snack: Apple Slices with Almond Butter

Ingredients: 1 apple, 2 tablespoons of almond butter.

Preparation: Slice the apple and serve with almond butter.

Dinner: Grilled Steak with Asparagus and Side Salad

Ingredients: 1 steak, 1 cup asparagus, 2 cups mixed greens, 1/2 cup cherry tomatoes, 1 tablespoon olive oil, 1 tablespoon balsamic vinegar, salt and pepper to taste.

Preparation: Grill the steak to desired doneness. Steam or grill asparagus. Toss mixed greens and cherry tomatoes with olive oil, balsamic vinegar, salt, and pepper.

Day 11:

Breakfast: Chia Seed Pudding with Coconut Milk and Fresh Berries

Ingredients: 1/4 cup chia seeds, 1 cup coconut milk, and 1/2 cup fresh berries.

Preparation: Mix chia seeds and coconut milk; refrigerate overnight. Top with fresh berries before serving.

Lunch: Quinoa and Black Bean Salad with Cilantro and Lime Dressing

Ingredients: 1 cup cooked quinoa, 1 cup black beans, 1/2 cup corn, 1/2 cup cherry tomatoes, 1/4 cup cilantro, 1 tbsp. olive oil, 1 tbsp. lime, salt, and pepper to taste.

Preparation: Mix quinoa, black beans, corn, cherry tomatoes, and cilantro. Dress with oil, lime juice, salt, and pepper.

Snack: Mixed Nuts

Ingredients: 1/4 cup mixed nuts.

Dinner: Baked Cod with Sautéed Kale and Sweet Potato Mash

Ingredients: 1 cod fillet, 1 cup kale, 1 sweet potato, 1 tablespoon olive oil, pepper, and salt to taste.

Preparation: Preheat oven to 375°F (190°C). Season cod fillet with salt and pepper, then bake for 15-20 minutes. Sauté kale in olive oil until wilted. Boil sweet potato, mash, and season with salt and pepper.

Day 12:

Breakfast: Ouellette with Tomatoes, Mushrooms, and Spinach

Ingredients: 2 eggs, 1/2 cup diced tomatoes, 1/2 cup sliced mushrooms, 1 cup spinach, salt and pepper to taste.

Preparation: Whisk eggs and pour into a heated pan. Add tomatoes, mushrooms, and spinach. Cook until eggs are set.

Lunch: Chicken Caesar Salad (with Olive Oil and Lemon Dressing)

Ingredients: 1 chicken breast, 2 cups romaine lettuce, 1/4 cup grated Parmesan, 1 tbsp. olive oil, 1 tbsp. lemon juice, salt, and pepper to taste.

Preparation: Grill or bake chicken breast. Toss romaine lettuce, Parmesan, olive oil, lemon juice, salt, and pepper. Top with sliced chicken.

Snack: Bell Pepper Slices with Guacamole

Ingredients: 1 bell pepper, 1/4 cup guacamole.

Preparation: Slice bell pepper and serve with guacamole.

Dinner: Turkey Meatballs with Zucchini Noodles and Marinara Sauce

Ingredients: 1 lb. ground turkey, 1 egg, 1/4 cup almond flour, 1/4 cup grated Parmesan, 2 zucchinis, 1 cup marinara sauce, 1 tbsp. olive oil, salt, and pepper.

Preparation: Preheat oven to 375°F (190°C). Mix ground turkey, egg, almond flour, Parmesan, salt, and pepper. Form into balls, bake for 25 minutes. Spiralize zucchinis into noodles and sauté in olive oil for 3-5 minutes. Serve meatballs over zucchini noodles with marinara sauce.

Breakfast: Greek Yogurt with Walnuts and Honey

Ingredients: 1 cup Greek yogurt, 1/4 cup walnuts, 1 tbsp. honey.

Preparation: Top the Greek yogurt with walnuts and drizzle with honey.

Lunch: Mixed Greens with Grilled Chicken, Avocado, and Balsamic Vinaigrette

Ingredients: 1 chicken breast, 2 cups mixed greens, 1/2 avocado, 1 tbsp. olive oil, and 1 tbsp. balsamic vinegar, salt and pepper to taste.

Preparation: Grill or bake the chicken breast. Toss the mixed greens, avocado, olive oil, balsamic vinegar, salt, and pepper together. Top the salad with sliced chicken.

Snack: Blueberries and Dark Chocolate

Ingredients: 1/2 cup blueberries, 1 oz. dark chocolate (70% cacao or higher).

Dinner: Grilled Salmon with Roasted Brussels sprouts and Quinoa

Ingredients: 1 salmon fillet, 1 cup Brussels sprouts, 1 cup cooked quinoa, 1 tbsp. olive oil, salt and pepper to taste.

Preparation: Preheat the oven to 400°F (200°C). Toss the Brussels sprouts with olive oil, salt, and pepper, then roast for 20-25 minutes. Grill the salmon until cooked through and serve with quinoa.

Day 14:

Breakfast: Kale, Banana, Almond Butter, and Flaxseed Smoothie

Ingredients: 1 cup kale, 1 banana, 1 tbsp. almond butter, 1 tbsp. flaxseeds, 1 cup almond milk.

Preparation: Blend all ingredients together until smooth.

Lunch: Spinach and Feta Stuffed Bell Peppers

Ingredients: 2 bell peppers, 1 cup spinach, 1/2 cup feta cheese, 1 tbsp. olive oil, salt and pepper to taste.

Preparation: Preheat the oven to 375°F (190°C). Remove the seeds from the bell peppers. Sauté the spinach in olive oil until wilted, then mix it with feta cheese. Stuff the bell peppers with the spinach and feta mixture and bake for 20–25 minutes.

Snack: Pumpkin Seeds

Ingredients: 1/4 cup pumpkin seeds.

 Grilled Pork Chops with Green Beans and Mashed Cauliflower

Ingredients: 1 pork chop, 1 cup green beans, 1 head cauliflower, 1 tablespoon olive oil, salt and pepper to taste.

Preparation: Grill the pork chop to your desired doneness. Steam or sauté the green beans. Boil the cauliflower, mash it, and season with salt and pepper.

Day 15:

Breakfast: Greek Yogurt with Mixed Berries

Ingredients: 1 cup Greek yogurt, 1/2 cup mixed berries of different varieties

Preparation: Mix Greek yogurt with berries in a bowl and serve immediately.

Lunch: Grilled Chicken Salad with Avocado

Ingredients: 1 grilled chicken breast, 2 cups mixed greens, 1/2 avocado, 1 tbsp. olive oil, and 1 tbsp. balsamic vinegar

Preparation: Grill the chicken breast and slice it. Toss mixed greens with olive oil and balsamic vinegar, then top with sliced chicken and avocado.

Snack: Walnuts

Ingredients: 1/4 cup walnuts

Ingredients: 1 salmon fillet, 1 cup broccoli, 1 tbsp. olive oil, salt, and pepper

Preparation: Preheat oven to 375°F (190°C). Season the salmon with salt and pepper, bake for 15-20 minutes. Steam broccoli for 5-7 minutes.

Day 16:

Breakfast: **Spinach, Avocado, and Berry Smoothie**

Ingredients: 1 cup spinach, 1/2 avocado, 1/2 cup mixed berries, 1 cup almond milk

Preparation: Blend all ingredients until smooth.

Lunch: **Turkey and Avocado Lettuce Wraps**

Ingredients: 4 large lettuce leaves, 4 slices turkey breast, 1/2 avocado (sliced), 1 cup carrot sticks

Preparation: Place turkey and avocado on lettuce leaves, roll up, and secure with toothpicks. Serve with carrot sticks.

 Cucumber with Hummus

Ingredients: 1 cucumber, 1/4 cup hummus

Preparation: Slice cucumber and serve with hummus.

 Shrimp Stir-Fry

Ingredients: 1 lb. shrimp, 1 bell pepper (sliced), 1 zucchini (sliced), 1 cup quinoa, 2 tbsp. soy sauce

Preparation: Cook quinoa according to package instructions. Heat olive oil in a pan, add shrimp, bell pepper, and zucchini. Stir-fry shrimp until cooked and the vegetables are tender. Add soy sauce and serve over quinoa.

Day 17:

Breakfast: Scrambled Eggs with Tomatoes and Spinach

Ingredients: 2 eggs, 1/2 cup diced tomatoes, 1 cup spinach, salt, and pepper

Preparation: Sauté spinach and tomatoes in a pan until soft. Whisk eggs and pour over, cooking until scrambled.

Lunch: Tuna Salad with Mixed Greens

Ingredients: 1 can tuna, 2 cups mixed greens, 1/4 cup olives, 1 tablespoon olive oil, and 1 tablespoon of lemon juice

Preparation: Drain tuna and mix with olives. Toss the greens with olive oil and lemon. Serve tuna on top.

Snack: Apple with Almond Butter

Ingredients: 1 apple, 2 tbsp. almond butter

Preparation: Slice the apple and serve with almond butter.

Dinner: Grilled Steak with Asparagus

Ingredients: 1 steak, 1 cup asparagus, salt, and pepper

Preparation: Season steak with salt and pepper and grill to desired doneness. Steam or grill asparagus until tender.

Day 18:

Breakfast: Chia Seed Pudding

Ingredients: 1/4 cup chia seeds, 1 cup coconut milk, 1/2 cup berries

Preparation: Combine chia seeds and coconut milk, stir, and refrigerate overnight. Top with berries before serving.

Lunch: Quinoa and Black Bean Salad

Ingredients: 1 cup cooked quinoa, 1 cup black beans, 1/2 cup corn, 1/4 cup cilantro, 1 tablespoon. Lime juice

Preparation: Mix all ingredients in a bowl and serve chilled.

Ingredients: 1/4 cup mixed nuts

Dinner: Baked Cod with Sautéed Kale

Ingredients: 1 cod fillet, 1 cup kale, 1 sweet potato, 1 tablespoon olive oil

Preparation: Preheat oven to 375°F (190°C). Bake cod for 15-20 minutes. Sauté kale in olive oil until wilted. Boil sweet potato, mash, and serve alongside.

Breakfast: Omellette with Spinach and Feta

Ingredients: 2 eggs, 1 cup spinach, 1/4 cup feta cheese

Preparation: Whisk eggs, pour into a heated pan, and add spinach. Cook until set and sprinkle feta cheese before folding.

Lunch: Chicken Caesar Salad

Ingredients: 1 chicken breast, 2 cups romaine lettuce, 1/4 cup grated Parmesan, 1 tbsp. olive oil, 1 tbsp. lemon juice

Preparation: Grill chicken breast, slice, and toss with lettuce, Parmesan, olive oil, and lemon juice.

Snack: Bell Pepper with Guacamole

Ingredients: 1 bell pepper, 1/4 cup guacamole

Preparation: Slice bell pepper and serve with guacamole.

Dinner: Turkey Meatballs with Zucchini Noodles

Ingredients: 1 lb. ground turkey, 1 egg, 1/4 cup almond flour, 2 zucchinis, and 1 cup marinara sauce

Preparation: Preheat oven to 375°F (190°C). Mix turkey, egg, almond flour, salt, and pepper; form meatballs and bake for 20 minutes. Spiralize zucchinis, sauté, and serve with meatballs and marinara sauce.

Day 20:

Breakfast: Greek Yogurt with Walnuts and Honey

Ingredients: 1 cup Greek yogurt, 1/4 cup walnuts, 1 tablespoon honey

Preparation: Top Greek yogurt with walnuts and drizzle with honey.

Lunch: Mixed Greens with Grilled Chicken and Avocado

Ingredients: 1 chicken breast, 2 cups mixed greens, 1/2 avocado, 1 tablespoon balsamic vinaigrette

Preparation: Grill chicken, slice, and serve over mixed greens with avocado and dressing.

Snack: Blueberries and Dark Chocolate

Ingredients: 1/2 cup blueberries, 1 oz. dark chocolate

Dinner: Grilled Salmon with Brussels sprouts

Ingredients: 1 salmon fillet, 1 cup Brussels sprouts, 1 tablespoon olive oil

Preparation: Preheat oven to 400°F (200°C). Toss Brussels sprouts with olive oil, salt, and pepper, roast for 20 minutes. Grill salmon until cooked through.

Day 21:

Breakfast: Kale, Banana, Almond Butter, and Flaxseed Smoothie

Ingredients: 1 cup kale, 1 banana, 1 tbsp almond butter, 1 tbsp. flaxseeds, 1 cup almond milk

Preparation: Blend all ingredients until smooth.

Lunch: Spinach and Feta Stuffed Bell Peppers

Ingredients: 2 bell peppers, 1 cup spinach, and 1/2 cup feta cheese

Preparation: Preheat oven to 375°F (190°C).Remove the seeds from the pepper. Sauté spinach, mix with feta, stuff peppers, and bake for 20–25 minutes.

Snack: Pumpkin Seeds

Ingredients: 1/4 cup pumpkin seeds

 Grilled Pork Chops with Green Beans

Ingredients: 1 pork chop, 1 cup green beans, 1 head cauliflower

Preparation: Grill pork chop to desired doneness. Steam green beans. Boil cauliflower, mash, and season.

Day 22:

Breakfast: Greek Yogurt with Mixed Berries

Ingredients: 1 cup Greek yogurt, 1/2 cup mixed berries of different varieties

Preparation: Combine Greek yogurt and berries in a bowl and serve immediately.

Lunch: Grilled Chicken Salad with Avocado

Ingredients: 1 grilled chicken breast, 2 cups mixed greens, 1/2 avocado, 1 tbsp. olive oil, and 1 tbsp. balsamic vinegar

Preparation: Grill the chicken breast for 6-8 minutes per side. Slice and toss with mixed greens, olive oil, and balsamic vinegar. Top with sliced avocado.

Snack: Handful of Walnuts

Ingredients: 1/4 cup walnuts

 Baked Salmon with Steamed Broccoli

Ingredients: 1 salmon fillet, 1 cup broccoli, 1 tablespoon olive oil, salt, and pepper

Preparation: Preheat oven to 375°F (190°C). Season salmon with salt and pepper, place on a baking sheet, and bake for 15-20 minutes. Steam broccoli until tender to your choice, about 5-7 minutes.

Day 23:

Breakfast: Spinach, Avocado, and Berry Smoothie

Ingredients: 1 cup spinach, 1/2 avocado, 1/2 cup mixed berries, 1 cup almond milk

Preparation: Blend all ingredients until smooth. Serve immediately.

Lunch: Turkey and Avocado Lettuce Wraps

Ingredients: 4 large lettuce leaves, 4 slices turkey breast, 1/2 avocado (sliced), 1 cup carrot sticks

Preparation: Place turkey and avocado on lettuce leaves, roll up tightly, and secure with toothpicks. Serve with carrot sticks.

Snack: Sliced Cucumber with Hummus

Ingredients: 1 cucumber, 1/4 cup hummus

Preparation: Slice cucumber and serve with hummus.

Dinner: Shrimp Stir-Fry

Ingredients: 1 lb. shrimp, 1 bell pepper (sliced), 1 zucchini (sliced), 1 cup quinoa, 2 tbsp. soy sauce

Preparation: Cook quinoa as per package instructions. Heat olive oil in a skillet, cook shrimp until pink (about 3-4 minutes). Add bell pepper and zucchini, stir-fry until tender. Add soy sauce and mix well. Serve over quinoa.

Day 24:

Breakfast: Scrambled Eggs with Spinach and Feta

Ingredients: 2 eggs, 1 cup spinach, 1/4 cup feta cheese

Preparation: Sauté spinach until wilted. Whisk eggs, pour over spinach, and stir until cooked through. Add feta cheese and mix gently.

Lunch: Tuna Salad with Mixed Greens

Ingredients: 1 can tuna, 2 cups mixed greens, 1/4 cup olives, 1 tbsp. olive oil, and 1 tbsp. lemon juice

Preparation: Drain tuna and mix with olives. Toss the greens with olive oil and lemon juice. Serve tuna on top.

 Apple Slices with Almond Butter

Ingredients: 1 apple, 2 tbsp. almond butter

Preparation: Slice the apple and serve with almond butter.

 Grilled Steak with Asparagus

Ingredients: 1 steak, 1 cup asparagus, salt, and pepper

Preparation: Season steak with salt and pepper, grill to desired doneness (4-5 minutes per side for medium). Steam or grill asparagus until tender, about 5-7 minutes.

Day 25:

Breakfast: Chia Seed Pudding

Ingredients: 1/4 cup chia seeds, 1 cup coconut milk, 1/2 cup berries

Preparation: Combine chia seeds and coconut milk in a bowl, stir well, and refrigerate overnight. Top with berries in the morning.

Lunch: Quinoa and Black Bean Salad

Ingredients: 1 cup cooked quinoa, 1 cup black beans, 1/2 cup corn, 1/4 cup cilantro, 1 tbsp. lime juice

Preparation: Mix all ingredients in a bowl and serve chilled.

Snack: Mixed Nuts

Ingredients: 1/4 cup mixed nuts

Dinner: Baked Cod with Sautéed Kale

Ingredients: 1 cod fillet, 1 cup kale, 1 sweet potato, 1 tbsp. olive oil

Preparation: Preheat oven to 375°F (190°C). Bake cod for 15-20 minutes. Sauté kale in olive oil until wilted. Boil sweet potato until tender, mash, and serve with cod and kale.

Day 26:

Breakfast: Omelette with Tomatoes and Spinach

Ingredients: 2 eggs, 1/2 cup diced tomatoes, 1 cup spinach, salt, and pepper

Preparation: Whisk eggs with salt and pepper. Sauté spinach and tomatoes in a skillet. Pour eggs over vegetables and cook until set.

Lunch: Chicken Caesar Salad

Ingredients: 1 chicken breast, 2 cups romaine lettuce, 1/4 cup grated Parmesan, 1 tbsp. olive oil, 1 tbsp. lemon juice

Preparation: Grill chicken breast, slice, and toss with romaine, Parmesan, olive oil, and lemon juice.

Snack: Bell Pepper Slices with Guacamole

Ingredients: 1 bell pepper, 1/4 cup guacamole

Preparation: Slice bell pepper and serve with guacamole.

Dinner: Turkey Meatballs with Zucchini Noodles

Ingredients: 1 lb. ground turkey, 1 egg, 1/4 cup almond flour, 2 zucchinis, 1 cup marinara sauce

Preparation: Preheat oven to 375°F (190°C). Mix turkey, egg, almond flour, salt, and pepper; form meatballs and bake for 20 minutes. Spiralize zucchinis, sauté, and serve with meatballs and marinara sauce.

Day 27:

Breakfast: Greek Yogurt with Walnuts and Honey

Ingredients: 1 cup Greek yogurt, 1/4 cup walnuts, 1 tbsp honey

Preparation: Top Greek yogurt with walnuts and drizzle with honey.

Lunch: Mixed Greens with Grilled Chicken and Avocado

Ingredients: 1 chicken breast, 2 cups mixed greens, 1/2 avocado, 1 tbsp. balsamic vinaigrette

Preparation: Grill chicken breast, slice, and toss with mixed greens, avocado, and balsamic vinaigrette.

Snack: Blueberries and Dark Chocolate

Ingredients: 1/2 cup blueberries, 1 oz. dark chocolate

 Grilled Salmon with Brussels sprouts

Ingredients: 1 salmon fillet, 1 cup Brussels sprouts, 1 tbsp. olive oil

Preparation: Preheat oven to 400°F (200°C). Toss Brussels sprouts with olive oil, salt, and pepper, roast for 20 minutes. Grill salmon until cooked through.

Day 28:

Breakfast: Kale, Banana, Almond Butter, and Flaxseed Smoothie

Ingredients: 1 cup kale, 1 banana, 1 tbsp almond butter, 1 tbsp. flaxseeds, 1 cup almond milk

Preparation: Blend all ingredients until smooth. Serve immediately.

Lunch: Spinach and Feta Stuffed Bell Peppers

Ingredients: 2 bell peppers, 1 cup spinach, 1/2 cup feta cheese

Preparation: Preheat oven to 375°F (190°C). Remove the seeds from the pepper. Sauté spinach in olive oil until wilted. Mix with feta, stuff into peppers, and bake for 20–25 minutes.

Snack: Pumpkin Seeds

Ingredients: 1/4 cup pumpkin seeds

Dinner: Grilled Pork Chops with Green Beans

Ingredients: 1 pork chop, 1 cup green beans, 1 head cauliflower

Preparation: Grill pork chop to desired doneness. Steam green beans. Boil cauliflower until tender, mash, and season.

Day 29:

Breakfast: Chia Seed Pudding with Berries

Ingredients: 1/4 cup chia seeds, 1 cup coconut milk, 1/2 cup mixed berries

Preparation: Combine chia seeds and coconut milk in a large bowl. Stir well and refrigerate overnight. Top with berries before serving.

Lunch: Quinoa and Black Bean Salad

Ingredients: 1 cup cooked quinoa, 1 cup black beans, 1/2 cup corn, 1/4 cup cilantro, 1 tablespoon lime juice

Preparation: Mix all ingredients in a bowl and serve chilled.

Snack: Mixed Nuts

Ingredients: 1/4 cup mixed nuts

Dinner: Baked Cod with Sautéed Kale

Ingredients: 1 cod fillet, 1 cup kale, 1 sweet potato, 1 tbsp. olive oil

Preparation: Preheat oven to 375°F (190°C). Bake cod for 15-20 minutes. Sauté kale in olive oil until wilted. Boil sweet potato, mash, and serve with cod and kale.

Day 30:

Breakfast: Omelette with Spinach and Tomatoes

Ingredients: 2 eggs, 1 cup spinach, 1/2 cup diced tomatoes, salt, and pepper

Preparation: Sauté spinach and tomatoes in a skillet until soft. Whisk eggs and pour over the vegetables, cooking until set.

Lunch: Chicken Caesar Salad

Ingredients: 1 chicken breast, 2 cups romaine lettuce, 1/4 cup grated Parmesan, 1 tbsp. olive oil, 1 tbsp. lemon juice

Preparation: Grill chicken breast, slice, and toss with romaine, Parmesan, olive oil, and lemon juice.

Snack: Bell Pepper Slices with Guacamole

Ingredients: 1 bell pepper, 1/4 cup guacamole

Preparation: Slice bell pepper and serve with guacamole.

Dinner: Turkey Meatballs with Zucchini Noodles

Ingredients: 1 lb. ground turkey, 1 egg, 1/4 cup almond flour, 2 zucchinis, and 1 cup marinara sauce

Preparation: Preheat oven to 375°F (190°C). Mix turkey, egg, almond flour, salt, and pepper; form meatballs and bake for 20 minutes. Spiralize zucchinis, sauté, and serve with meatballs and marinara sauce.

This completes the **30-day** meal plan, with detailed preparation methods for each meal. Enjoy your journey on the Galveston Diet!

CHAPTER 8

Galveston Diet Glossary

1. Anti-Inflammatory Diet: A diet aimed at reducing body inflammation by consuming foods high in antioxidants, omega-3 fatty acids, and other beneficial nutrients.

2. Intermittent Fasting: An eating pattern that alternates between periods of eating and fasting, often used in the Galveston Diet for weight management and improved metabolic health.

3. Macronutrients: Essential nutrients needed in large quantities for energy and bodily functions, including carbohydrates, proteins, and fats.

4. Healthy Fats: Beneficial unsaturated fats that support heart health and overall wellness, found in foods like avocados, nuts, seeds, and olive oil.

5. Lean Proteins: Low-fat protein sources such as chicken, turkey, fish, legumes, and plant-based proteins.

6. Whole Foods: Minimally processed foods that are close to their natural state, such as fruits, vegetables, whole grains, nuts, and seeds.

7. Processed Foods: Foods altered from their natural state through manufacturing, often containing added sugars, unhealthy fats, and artificial ingredients.

8. Nutrient-Dense: Foods rich in vitamins, minerals, and other beneficial nutrients relative to their calorie content.

9. Fiber: A type of carbohydrate found in plant foods that aids digestion and promotes a healthy gut.

10. Omega-3 Fatty Acids: Essential fatty acids with anti-inflammatory properties found in fish, flaxseeds, chia seeds, and walnuts, which benefit heart health.

11. Phytonutrients: Health-promoting natural compounds found in plants, including antioxidants and anti-inflammatory agents.

12. Hydration: Maintaining adequate fluid levels in the body, crucial for overall health and proper bodily functions.

13. Satiety: The feeling of fullness and satisfaction after eating, which helps control appetite and prevent overeating.

14. Glycemic Index: A measure of how quickly a food raises blood sugar levels. The Galveston Diet focuses on foods with a low glycemic index to manage blood sugar.

15. Hormone Balance: The regulation and balance of hormones in the body, impacting weight, mood, and overall health.

16. Metabolic Health: Having optimal levels of blood sugar, blood pressure, cholesterol, and other indicators, reducing the risk of chronic diseases.

17. Inflammation: The body's response to injury or infection, which can become chronic and lead to health issues if not managed.

18. Meal Planning: Organizing and preparing meals in advance to ensure a balanced and nutritious diet.

19. Portion Control: Managing the amount of food consumed in one sitting to maintain a healthy weight and prevent overeating.

20. Clean Eating: A dietary approach that emphasizes whole, minimally processed foods and avoids artificial ingredients and additives.

These terms cover the key concepts and components of the Galveston Diet, providing a foundational understanding for anyone interested in this dietary approach.

CHAPTER 9

CONCLUSION

In summary, the Galveston Diet presents a powerful pathway to improved health and wellness, enabling you to take charge of your dietary decisions and enhance your overall quality of life. By focusing on whole foods, practicing mindful eating, and incorporating intermittent fasting, you can effectively manage your weight, decrease inflammation, and enhance metabolic health. This approach goes beyond mere dieting; it represents a fundamental lifestyle change that nurtures balance, energy, and resilience. As you begin this journey, keep in mind that true change comes through dedication and consistency. Embrace the Galveston Diet principles, and discover the potential for a healthier, happier version of yourself—beginning now. Your future self will be grateful!

* 9 7 9 8 3 3 5 8 3 4 6 6 7 *